The Power of Eucalyptus for Health & Healing

by

Jack Malloy

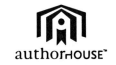

authorHOUSE™

1663 LIBERTY DRIVE, SUITE 200
BLOOMINGTON, INDIANA 47403
(800) 839-8640
WWW.AUTHORHOUSE.COM

First published by AuthorHouse 01/11/05

ISBN: 1-4208-1495-8 (sc)

Printed in the United States of America
Bloomington, Indiana

This book is printed on acid-free paper.

Table of Contents

Introduction

People have used plants, herbs and other natural remedies for thousands of years to help keep healthy and to heal themselves. This tradition has been found in every civilization and culture throughout human history. Only in the last century did pharmaceutical drugs take over in the industrial countries as the primary approach to treat disease. In some cases, drugs are appropriate, but not in all cases. As we rediscover nature's medicine chest through the work of modern research, a whole new world of therapies opens to us... **natural therapies.** These can be used to not only heal, but to strengthen and enhance our quality of life.

These natural therapies are often as effective as pharmaceutical drugs, but without the side effects. Many medicinal plants contain properties to heal that no synthetic drug has been able to mimic. This book is about one such plant...Eucalyptus. I wish not to bore you with complicated, technical and sometimes conflicting medical research data; although I have included a few studies. I do want to present a common sense understanding of how you can use eucalyptus oil to improve your health. Eucalyptus has been known for centuries as "Nature's Tree of Life". There is good reason for this accolade. I have introduced eucalyptus oil to thousands of people who have successfully used it to treat a variety of ailments. I get a great deal of pleasure hearing from them, some of their success stories are in this publication. I am confident you will appreciate these inspirational accounts just as I have. After reading this book, it is my hope you use this information to improve your health as it has mine.

Chapter One

Eucalyptus, A History of Healing

The name eucalyptus is derived from the Greek eu, meaning 'well', and kalyptos, meaning 'cover'. Eu Kalyptos refers to the well-covered flower buds, which are cone shaped and have a lid-like structure that opens as the flowers mature. Over the years as the medicinal benefits became apparent this meaning has been expanded to mean that eucalyptus "covers well" a variety of common conditions.

Over 600 Species of Eucalyptus

All eucalyptus trees originate in Australia. The 600 or so species have been transplanted to many other warm parts of the world such as Central Asia, North Africa, and parts of the warmer climates of Europe, North and South America. The trees are fast growing and are beautifully picturesque. Not only are they esthetic to the eye, they serve well to prevent soil erosion and provide a welcome home for a number of unique and endangered critters.

The evergreen eucalyptus tree's bark can exude a sweet smelling gum. However, the leaves contain droplets of essential oil and those of the Tasmanian Blue Gum are considered the most esteem for healing.

Historians tell us the Aborigines of Australia relied on this native evergreen for soothing painful joints and healing skin lesions. Settlers to the continent dubbed it the "Fever Tree" in recognition of its disease-fighting powers.

Once Europeans were introduced to the eucalyptus tree, they too rapidly recognized its gifts, medicinal and otherwise. In fact, they began to rely so heavily on eucalyptus oil for sterilizing medical and surgical equipment that it was briefly referred to as "catheter oil". Referring to the oil's ability to purge bacteria and sterilize.

Early Eucalyptus Studies

Oil of eucalyptus has been distilled since at least 1788 when two doctors, John White and Dennis Cossiden, distilled eucalyptus for its use in treating chest problems and colic. Early works on the antiseptic and bacterial properties of the oil were published in Germany by Dr. Colez (1870). This was followed by a publication by Dr. Faust and Dr. Homeyer in 1874. They classified it as being sudorific, anticatarrhal and astringent. It was prescribed for all respiratory system conditions such as bronchitis, flu, asthma and coughs.

As the use of eucalyptus spread, history records many more applications. In parts of Asia, travelers used it as a topical liniment. It's especially soothing for tired sore feet and muscles. Combined with other essential oils, it traditionally is used throughout South and Central America to ease the pain of arthritis and other muscle, ligament and tendon afflictions. Researchers document its effectiveness for respiratory infections, sinus headaches, flu, chicken pox, measles and herpes. Aborigines favored its use for fever reduction. Its stimulating effects aid in circulation and reduce muscle tension. Aborigine messengers would inhale eucalyptus vapors to enhance their lung capacity prior to running ten to thirty miles when delivering messages between villages.

Eucalyptus to the Rescue

An insightful story comes down through the ages which took place in central Australia about an arranged marriage between the son and the daughter of the leaders of warring clans. As the legend goes...these two villages had been on bad terms for as long as anyone could remember. There were many wars and much bloodshed. The son of the leader of one of the villages and the daughter of the leader of the rival village had come of age to marry. They were both about fourteen years old. A politically astute wise man of one of the villages saw this as an opportunity to arrange a marriage which would finally bring peace to the entire region. The marriage was arranged, a date was set. Hopefully, there would be no more wars and bloodshed.

As was the tradition, the family of the groom arrived in the village of the bride about ten days before the date of the marriage ceremony. This was a marriage of royalty. Agreements had to be made and boundaries had to be restructured so a lasting peace could take place. It was done and all were looking forward to years of harmony. The groom was left home with three or four advisors to prepare this child for married life. The groom was to arrive only on the day of the wedding to meet his bride for the first time.

The villages were about fifty miles apart. Three days prior to the wedding date the groom and his advisers set out on pack animals for the bride's village. They needed to arrive the day of the wedding at the time when the sun was highest in the sky. They planned the trip well. They took plenty of food and water and were well prepared for the journey. They could not be late. If the groom did not arrive on time, the bride's family would consider it the ultimate insult and would slaughter the groom's entire family.

A day into their journey, they were attacked by a roving clan of outlaws. The groom's advisors were all killed and he was left for dead. That evening the boy regained consciousness with a severe wound across his head. He had lost much blood and was weak and confused. The food, water and all the pack animals had been stolen. It looked hopeless, but the boy was determined to get to his bride's village. The boy saw a grove of eucalyptus trees in the distance and headed toward them. He knew he could rely on the healing power of eucalyptus leaves to prevent infection and to regain his strength. He had probably thirty five miles to go and only a day and a half to do it. He had to get there on time and he had to do it on foot. The lives of his entire family depended on it. He wrapped his head in eucalyptus leaves. He had known since a baby to inhale the vapors of eucalyptus to improve breathing. He took a handful of leaves and twisted them in his hands and held them close to his nose. The refreshing aroma cleared his head. He became even more focused now on the task ahead. He started running, taking with him only a few handfuls of eucalyptus leaves. He ran and ran and ran, stopping only to refresh himself with another breath of eucalyptus.

The wedding day had arrived. The sun was high above. The families were gathered. The ceremony was ready to begin and out from the forest the groom came running. His wound bloody, but not infected. He held a few leaves of eucalyptus in his hand which he twisted together and quickly took a long relaxing breath and proudly announced "I'm here to be married". The ceremony began on time and the couple was married as arranged. The bride and the groom went off to a specially prepared hut to consummate the marriage. Some time later the bride came running out of the hut screaming. The boy had collapsed from exhaustion. As the legend goes...no one is sure if he succumbed from exhaustion because of his wound, the run or his honeymoon. In any event, the marriage joined the two territories. The villages remained friendly from that point on.

A eucalyptus tree was planted to commemorate the strength of this union and the young boy's commitment. All future clan meetings and ceremonies were then conducted in the shade of this extraordinary tree.

The Australian folklore is rich with stories like this one. Some are funny and some are meant to convey a lesson. All of them reflect how eucalyptus touched their lives and became a part of their history.

The Lizard Family of Asia

In part of Eastern Asia eucalyptus has been traditionally used in a hot bath for those who suffered from colds, flu, sore muscles, exhaustion and stress. Historical accounts in Asia document a tradition of using eucalyptus in a weekly bath to rid the body of mites and other parasites. Its antiseptic action on the skin does wonders for sores and numerous other skin irritations.

There's an interesting story of a family in China who were known as the "lizard family." This was a large family that included cousins and other relatives. As the members of this family grew to adulthood they would develop a debilitating skin condition. Their skin would get dry and crack. In some cases the cracking wound would bleed. This was a chronic condition that would eventually cover their entire body. After years of continued cracking and bleeding, the skin would discolor leaving the person with dark scaly skin resembling a lizard. A visitor from "across the sea" came to see this family and brought with him eucalyptus leaves. He covered the arm of one of the afflicted men with a branch of eucalyptus and told him to leave it there until he returned in a few days. On his next visit he was greeted by the entire "lizard family". The arm where the eucalyptus was wrapped had almost completely healed. More eucalyptus was brought. They boiled it in water and poured the oil into a bath. The whole family used it and over time they all recovered. Eucalyptus saplings were planted and a new part of the world came to know the benefits of eucalyptus.

Eucalyptus is truly one of nature's great gifts. Accounts such as these can be found in the history of almost every civilization. Every culture that has had the good fortune to be exposed to it has embraced it. It has stood the test of time. Modern research is now rediscovering the full benefits of eucalyptus.

The Many Uses of Eucalyptus

In the years I have worked with eucalyptus liniment through introducing it to thousands of people, I am always pleasantly surprised when I hear from those who tell me about new uses for this remarkable oil. Listed here are some of the applications. No doubt there are many more. Some of these uses are covered more thoroughly in this book and some will be expanded as research continues to uncover the many applications of this extraordinary gift from nature.

- Eucalyptus oil expands alveoli (tiny air sacs in the lungs), temporarily expanding lung capacity.
- It increases air flow into the lungs and increases oxygen flow to the body.
- Eucalyptus coats the airways and sloughs off all infected mucosal surfaces leaving the cold and virus germs with nowhere to take hold.
- Effects are nearly immediate.
- It acts as a decongestant, reduces nasal dripping, reduces nasal stuffiness and helps to clear sinuses.
- It reduces the severity of sinusitis.
- It can prevent asthma attacks.
- Has been used to treat asthma and reduces the severity of asthma attacks.
- It can reduce the severity of some respiratory allergies.
- It thins mucus in nasal passages.
- It thins the mucus in bronchial passages.
- It thins the mucus in lungs and thus reduces the chances of getting lung infections.
- It is a good expectorant.
- It can reduce coughing.
- It is good for treating chronic bronchitis.
- It helps to clear mucus from obstructed "smoker's lungs".
- It helps to clear up raspy chest coughs.
- It's used to treat whooping coughs.

- It can prevent colds and flu.
- Reduces the severity of colds and flu.
- It can help to prevent the spread of head colds and flu into pneumonia.
- It kills infectious bacteria that can cause pneumonia.
- It is an antiviral.
- It is an antifungal.
- It kills certain antibiotic resistant pathogens.
- It kills dust mites. Many people with asthma are allergic to allergens from house dust mites.
- Good for treating COPD ("Chronic Obstructive Pulmonary Disease").
- It's an old time prescription for emphysema by preventing lung infections.
- It helps to improve circulation.
- It helps to expand blood vessels bringing more oxygen and nutrients to muscles, tendons and other soft tissue.
- It can reduce or prevent headaches and migraines.
- It helps to ease the pain of arthritis.
- It reduces muscle tension.
- The vapors are invigorating and help to improve concentration.
- It's an antiseptic for the skin.
- Its antiseptic action is good for cuts, burns, insect bites and other skin irritations.
- It's relaxing and soothing in a bath.

Testimonial

Sore stiff fingers feel great

I am an accountant and have arthritis in my fingers. Sometimes the pain is so bad that I cannot even hold a pencil and that is a big problem, especially during tax time.

I saw your display while I was in Atlantic City and tried a sample because my fingers were hurting so bad. The pain subsided a little immediately and the salesperson explained that was a good sign and by using it a couple times a day the results would continue to improve. It's now been about three weeks and my sore, stiff fingers feel great. I use it once a day and my fingers continue to improve. I have recommended this product to other accountants who suffer from the same ailment as I did.

Keven L.
Harrisburg, Pa.

Testimonial

Improved breathing for 10K run

I am an avid health nut. I'm always looking for natural ways to improve my body. I've read about the use of eucalyptus oil to improve breathing capacity and ordered your product to try it. I'm reporting back to let you know it really works.

I started breathing in the eucalyptus vapors while training for a 10 k run.

Last week I ran the event and improved my time by over two minutes.

Thanks, I will continue to keep you informed.

Danny B.
Los Angeles, California

Testimonial

Great for massage

I use your eucalyptus liniment in my massage studio. My customers love the fragrance and I'm especially pleased because the oil is very light and helps to improve circulation and adds to the overall positive effect of the massage.

Sincerely,

June A.

Salem, New Jersey

Chapter Two

Colds and Flu

Colds and flu are normally viral illnesses, commonly rhino viruses of which there are several thousand types. These are airborne microbes that lodge in the warm, moist membranes of the nasal and sinus passages. They form colonies there that can double in size every twenty minutes.

The medical treatment for this is generally antihistamines, decongestants and cough suppressants. These are all treatments for the symptoms of the infection, but very little treatment is directed toward the cause of the cold. Bed rest, keeping warm and plenty of fluids is still recognized as a common sense treatment. Sometimes antibiotics are used, even though we know that antibiotics never work on viruses. Rhino-virus infections normally last about three to four days. During this time the virus causes damage to the lining of the respiratory tract. Then, bacteria, which may be susceptible to antibiotics, move into the damaged tissue and set up secondary infections. These cause the yellow discharge of infected material from the nose that can last for weeks. Antibiotics are then used to kill the bacteria responsible for this secondary infection.

Doctor Says "Come back when you're sicker."

An old adage was that if you asked your doctor to help with your cold, he would say he couldn't. However, if you ignored it and came back a few days later with pneumonia, he could cure that with a shot of penicillin. The penicillin was effective in treating the bacteria responsible for the onset of pneumonia.

Prior to World War II antibiotics were not available. A frequent sequence in the pre antibiotic era was first cold, then pneumonia, then death. Colds were considered much more serious. Today people do die of pneumonia even with the use of antibiotics. Bacteria once completely wiped out by antibiotics have adapted and new forms are becoming common. The overuse of antibiotics has greatly accelerated the development of antibiotic resistant strains of disease parthenogenesis.

Antibiotics were given out like candy. They were so successful that they became the first rung of treatment. The public demanded a pill or shot and the pharmaceutical companies and the medical profession were more than willing to supply it. Most germs are now not affected by older antibiotics, and some are not affected by any antibiotics now available. The old cycle is making a come back. Colds go to pneumonia which may not be cured by a shot or a pill. Deaths due to antibiotic resistant pneumonia and other bacteria diseases are on the increase. Antibiotics, had they only been used as a back up to prevent serious consequences, might have eluded bacterial adaptation for some centuries. So maybe it is time to look at some old proven treatments that have been used through the ages that are not dependent on antibiotics.

Eucalyptus Inhibits Bacterial and Viral Growth

Eucalyptus oil is a natural, broad-spectrum anti-microbial. It effectively inhibits growth of bacteria and viral replication. Inhaling eucalyptus coats the respiratory tract forming a protective layer which sheds off, taking any viruses with it.

A particularly relevant publication entitled **"Antibacterial Activity of Essential Oils and Their Major Constituents Against Respiratory Tract Pathogens By Gaseous Contact"** written by Shigeharu Inouye, Toshio Takizawa and Hideyo Yamaguchi that was published in ***The Journal of Antimicrobial Chemotherapy*** in 2001 (The British Society for Antimicrobial Chemotherapy) confirms the effectiveness of eucalyptus vapors and other essential oils against a variety of ailments.

This publication states in part the following: *"The antibacterial activity of 14 essential oils and their major constituents in the gaseous state was evaluated against Haemophilus, Streptococcus pneumoniae, (a disease related to the lungs), Streptococcus pyogenes, (fever producing illness) and Staphylococcus aureus, (related to the ear or sense of hearing). For most essential oils H. influenzae was most susceptible, followed by S. pneumoniae and S. pyogenes, and then S. aureus."* It further states, *"These results indicate that the antibacterial action of essential oils was most effective when at high vapor concentration for a short time."* This study continues to state, *"Essential oils produced by plants have been traditionally used for respiratory tract infections, and are used nowadays as ethical medicines for colds. In the medicinal field, inhalation therapy of essential oils has been used to treat acute and chronic bronchitis and acute sinusitis. Inhalation of vapors of essential oils augmented the output of respiratory tract fluid, maintained the ventilation and drainage of the sinuses, had anti-inflammatory effect on the trachea and reduced asthma."* The study goes on to document the effectiveness of eucalyptus for its antiviral and antifungal properties.

Use Eucalyptus to Treat and Prevent Colds and Flu

The simplicity of this is obvious. During the cold and flu season, spray a little eucalyptus oil liniment on the palms of your hands, then cup your hands near your nose and inhale through your nose and exhale out of your mouth three times. Do this about once a day. It's refreshing and this kind of natural prevention helps to maintain an infection-free environment in your nasal passages and lungs. We are exposed to thousands of different types of viruses and bacteria daily. Your healthy immune system should destroy these viruses and the cells they invade before any symptoms develop.

In a healthy body this occurs routinely. Unfortunately, the overuse of drugs such as antibiotics actually impedes this natural defense from being as effective as it should be. We now have millions of people whose natural defenses are so devastated by these drugs that the slightest exposure leaves them sick and infected.

This weakened immune system, because of the overuse of antibiotics, also has a devastating effect on your normal colonic bacteria. It opens the door for a B12 deficiency which is made by the normal bacteria in the colon. This creates an opportunity for the invasion of Candida or other pathogens unless you deliberately restore these normal microbes. Antibiotics devastate good bacteria, as well as bad bacteria. The necessary digestive bacterial in the intestinal tract, that is vital for adsorption of nutrients, is highly sensitive and can be destroyed by antibiotics, leaving the person's digestive system with a diminished ability to absorb nutrients. At a time when you need all the nutrients you can get, your digestive system can't absorb them. There are few doctors who recommend eating yogurt or taking acidophilus (acidophilus helps to restore a supportive environment in the intestinal tract) when prescribing antibiotics as a treatment.

The best way to deal with colds and flu is by not getting in a condition where they can take hold in the first place. Stay healthy by living healthy. The key to that means enough exercise daily, good eating habits (that is a topic for another book) and taking personal responsibility for your health. Taking advantage of natural eucalyptus oil and other gifts from nature, as a preventative measure is easy to do and makes common sense. If you do get under the weather, employ the natural remedies as the first line of treatment. When your immune system is not devastated by the invasive use of drugs, your body responds faster and better. If you do get a cold or flu, you will find its duration is shorter and less severe.

I've spoken with many people who tell me they get colds and flu easily. They just get over one cold and then catch another one. I ask them, what are they doing about it? They tell me they take an over the counter medication for a while and then when that doesn't work they go to the doctor and get a prescription. This declining cycle goes on because the treatment they used left them in a more susceptible condition for the next infection. It seems to me that when you find the real reason for this cycle it should open the door for a solution. Well, the real "why" is not they have a shortage of antibiotics in their body. The real "why" is they have not maintained a healthy enough immune system. Living life to the fullest is an art form. Maintaining a healthy body takes a little knowledge, responsibility and just plain common sense. Using eucalyptus oil as a preventative measure is a simple and effective way to assist your immune system. These are things that can be done with just a little bit of attention in the right place. With the use of gifts from nature, I believe we can successfully prevent 90% of the illnesses currently taking up most of the doctor's time.

Testimonial

"I would be sick all the time"

I wanted to write to you to thank you for your eucalyptus liniment. About two years ago we moved from Dallas, Texas to Chicago. Even since I arrive here I've been sick with colds almost continuously. I took over the counter medicine and then antibiotics and as soon as I got over one cold I got another one. I was at the end of my rope and was ready to move back to Dallas.

My cousin gave me a bottle of the eucalyptus liniment and told me to spread some on my hands and inhale the vapors twice a day. I started to do that and with in two days my cold was gone. I couldn't believe it worked so fast. I continue to inhale the vapors at least once a day, especially during the cold winter months.

What a relief it is not to be sick all the time. I'm finally beginning to enjoy Chicago. Thank you for your life saving eucalyptus.

Jan P.
Chicago, Illinois

Testimonial

Sinus pain and headache were unbearable

For years I suffered from severe sinus congestion. The pain and the headaches were at times unbearable. I tried every medication I could find but nothing worked for long. I even became addicted to nose spray. I have a high presser job and could not afford to be side tracked by this sinus problem. So I just suffered through it, doing the best that I could, resigned to the fact that this was a condition for life and I would have to live with it.

A friend of mine at work saw me in a miserable state one day. I had a headache, my sinuses were completely blocked and I was feeling terrible. She sprayed a little of your eucalyptus liniment on the back of my neck and had me breath some of the eucalyptus vapors from a cotton ball. Almost immediately I could breathe better. A short time later my headache was gone. I was shocked. How could something this simple be so effective? I felt good the rest of the day. I bought a bottle and use it when needed and my sinuses are clear.

Many Thanks,
Joseph K.
Philadelphia, Pennsylvania

Testimonial

Day care worker, no longer gets flu

Just a short note to let you know I've used your eucalyptus liniment for about three years as a preventative measure against colds. I work at a day care center and during the cold and flu season many of our kids would be sick and I would always catch the germs and get sick myself. I like to use natural remedies and read how eucalyptus is a natural anti viral and anti bacterial and I wanted to do something to keep from getting sick from the germs. I started using your eucalyptus liniment by spraying it on my hands and breathing in the vapors daily. I'm happy to let you know I've not been sick since I started doing that, three years ago. Some of my coworkers are doing the same and they have had similar results.

Some of our parents now use your eucalyptus oil also. I hope you will pass this message to others who work in day care centers. It's always best to use a natural remedy, especially around children.

Thank You,
Martha T.
Baltimore, Maryland

Chapter Three

Infections and Skin Irritations

Eucalyptus is nature's strongest natural antiseptic. It originally was used in Australia to treat skin liaisons thereby preventing infections and improving the rate of recovery time. Those who use it just knew it worked and was effective. Now, modern research has uncovered the science behind it. Eucalyptus oil is perhaps one of nature's most versatile essential oils. Its effectiveness can be enhanced when combined with other essential oils.

Essential Oils Work When Antibiotics Fail

A recent study was reported in Dallas Texas about eucalyptus oil, combined with tea tree oil to combat infection. This was reported in Reuters Health and was entitled "Essential Oils Found to Fight Bacteria". The report states: *A pair of orthopedic surgeons report two essential oils...Eucalyptus and Tea Tree oil...are surprisingly effective at treating methicillin resistant Staphylocoous aureus (MRSA) infections.*

The researchers presented their findings in Dallas at the 69th Annual Meeting of the American Academy of Orthopedic Surgeons.

Dr. Eugene Sherry of the University of Sydney in Australia said that, applied to the skin of infected wounds an antibacterial was derived from Eucalyptus radiate and Melaleuca alternifonia, best known as Eucalyptus and Tea Tree, can work when modern antibiotics fail.

Dr. Sherry said that he used the combination "once a day for several months" in a series of 25 patients with MRSA. "Twenty-two of the infections resolve completely." Sherry reported. In 19 patients, the infections resolved without the use of antibiotics, while three patients required antibiotic treatment, he said.

Sixteen of the infections involved the bone and three had spread to muscle. In addition, 10 of the patients were diabetic, which" makes healing of wounds very difficult," Sherry said in an interview with Reuters Health.

Two years earlier, Dr. Sherry attended a presentation about the antibacterial properties of essential oils and decided to research the subject. He said that he discovered a wealth of 50 year old research concerning essential oils, but said, *"all that research was abandoned when modern science discovered antibiotics."*

When Dr. Sherry decided to initiate a trial of eucalyptus and tea tree oil in MRSA patients, he discovered that Dr. Patrick H. Warnke, an orthopedic surgeon at the University of Liel in Germany, was pursuing a parallel study; so the two combined their work to produce the 25 patient MRSA study.

Warnke said they are now studying an aerosolized version of the compound in laboratory studies of tuberculosis. When they sprayed the compound on tuberculosis cultures *"We wiped out TB, killed it, in 40 minutes. No antibiotic does that,"* Warnke told Reuter Health.

Both doctors said that they have received no funding from the makers of essential oils, nor do they have financial interests in companies producing the substances. We are starting to see more of this kind of research but don't look for any great announcements about the success of these compounds from the pharmaceutical industry. These compounds are natural and are available to everyone now. They are not subject to patent protection and therefore the pharmaceutical industry can not position itself as financial benefactors from its use. The rediscovery of the benefits of essential oils is only in response to the current failures of the pharmaceutical solutions.

Remarkable Results with Eucalyptus Liniment

I have used eucalyptus oil combined with grape seed oil, aloe vera oil and jojoba oil and just a touch of vitamin E to help people treat a wide variety of skin irritations. You need not be a doctor to help people when they need assistance. I have seen remarkable results when this eucalyptus based liniment was applied to cuts, sores and abrasions. The oil successfully cleaned the wound, disinfected it, helped the wound heal and minimized scaring. It's wonderful for cold sores. In fact if you apply a drop or two to the cold sore before it erupts on the surface, the penetrating action of the oil will neutralize the infection before it reaches the surface.

I have seen outstanding results for rashes, insect bites, psoriasis, poison ivy and eczema. It is also great for burns and sunburn.

Testimonial

Had eczema all her life

I wanted to write to you to let you know what your eucalyptus liniment has done for me. I have had severe Eczema all my life. I have been to several doctors including specialists. I was told there was not much more they could do and I would have to learn to live with it. The Eczema continued to spread and now covered parts of my arms and shoulders and was starting on my face. I tried every product I could find but nothing really worked.

Finally, a friend of mine showed me your eucalyptus liniment. I half heartedly spread some on one of my arms and forgot about it. I had been disappointed so many times before that I had little faith that anything would do any good. Several hours later, I noticed the itching had stopped on that arm and the rash was less red and flaky. I called my friend and got your phone number off the bottle and the next day called and ordered a bottle.

I have now used your liniment for about a month and am happy to report my Eczema is almost totally gone. The few remaining spots are far less severe and I'm sure they will be gone also in time. I can now wear short sleeve shirts. Thank you.

Dorothy M.
Columbia, Maryland

Testimonial

"My friends can't keep up with me now"

I am 65 years old and I am a walker. My friends and I walk in the mall every morning for exercise. Each day we do several loops totaling about two miles. Six months ago my feet began to hurt from corns that were growing between my toes. I tried some over the counter remedies but nothing really helped. I saw my doctor and he told me that I would eventually have to have surgery to get them removed. I was not looking forward to that. I had difficulty keeping up with my friends while walking and could only complete half the loop because my feet were hurting so bad.

I saw your display of eucalyptus liniment and was desperate to try anything. I bought a bottle and started to use it each day on my feet. I was surprised because from the first day I had less pain in my feet. After a week, I noticed the corns were softening and starting to go away. I was overjoyed. My corns are now completely gone and I am doing the entire two mile loop again. My friends are having a hard time keeping up with me. Thank you so much for your all natural eucalyptus liniment. Please share my success story with others. I want all senior citizens to know there is a natural way they can keep up with their busy life.

Sincerely,

Betty B.

Dover, Delaware

Chapter Four

Natural Vasodilator

One of the exceptional properties of eucalyptus oil is its ability to improve circulation. Cineole, the active component in eucalyptus oil, activates the nerve cells surrounding the blood vessels causing them to relax and in so doing, helps to dilate the blood vessels. This action adds more oxygen and nutrients to the affected area. Eucalyptus can be categorized as a natural "vasodilator".

Much of the research about eucalyptus oil is done in Europe and Asia because the use of natural remedies is more widespread and traditional. An article published in the *Indian Journal of Pharmacology* about the effects of eucalyptus oil on capillary permeability addresses the issue of vasodilation. The article states: *"The leaf extract or essential oil from the leaves of eucalyptus species has been reported to possess antifungal, antibacterial, mosquito repellent and antioxidant properties.* The article goes on to say, *increased capillary permeability, at the site of a wound facilitates the healing process and that this essential oil produced an increase in vascular capillary permeability.*

This article goes on to quote a conclusion from an accompanying study: *The Vascular permeability-increasing action coupled with the reported antifungal, antibacterial and anti-inflammatory-analgesic effects of this essential oil may be highly beneficial for the promotion of wound healing.*

This increase in vascular permeability simply means the blood vessels are more open for passage. They are more open for blood flow. As a result, the body is more able to heal itself. Eucalyptus oil helps the body to heal itself.

Residual effect of Injuries

Injuries to any part of the body create a residual effect on circulation in that particular area. When the nerves sense an intrusion, such as a shock, trauma or other stress, the nerves around the blood vessels will create a muscular reaction surrounding the blood vessels causing a compression in the size of the blood vessel itself. This restricts blood flow to the area is the body's innate defense against bleeding to death. If you were to cut your arm and examine the blood vessels in that region, you would find an attempt to restrict the blood flow through the constriction of blood vessels. This pro-survival mechanism has undoubtedly saved the lives of numerous people. However, this superb defense mechanism can create residual long term debilitating conditions that can unduly influence proper circulation function in that area for the rest of the person's life.

Shortly after an injury has occurred the healing process starts. Nutrients, oxygen and other compounds are ushered to the injured area. The blood picks up damaged cells, cell waste and other elements and removes them from the vicinity. This process is continuous and to a less accentuated degree occurs non stop for every moment of life. After the injury has fully healed, the blood vessels then return to their normal size and regular function resumes.

Cells retain a lasting trace of injury

On many occasions the cells in the injured area retain a lasting trace of the injury. It's an actual memory of the injury. This is especially true if the shock of the injury caused some degree of unconsciousness. There is a great deal of research that validates this phenomenon. The connection between the individual's consciousness and his communication and control of his body is a vital factor in the seriousness of the injury, as well as, the speed of the healing process. This data has opened the door to remarkable results in the healing arena. This lasting trace residual memory is actually a stimulus response mechanism that triggers a future reaction when that area of the body is again threatened with stress or strain. During times when the individual is tired or under pressure those cells interpret that as a threat and react the same as they did during the original injury. The nerves are quick to respond by compressing the blood vessels again and again. It's as if the cells in the injured area get stuck in time. They are in a constant state of tension. They continually relive the injury. Even though the injury will heal, the cells to a greater or lesser degree still experience the injury. They are stuck in the injury and continue to react as if they are constantly at that moment. Time moves forward, life continues and the full function of the damaged area is handicapped by the cellular memory of a long gone injury. The body should repair itself after an injury with little to no residual effect. The lasting trace inhibits this process and accounts for life long debilitating aches and pains.

This scenario plays out hundreds of times in a person's life. As a result, full circulation may never return to the injured area for long. It is my guess that this is more the rule than the exception.

This same process also occurs in parts of the body where there was no specific injury. Continuous stress from poor posture, or spending numerous hours hovering over a computer can, over time, generate the same effect on he body's circulation system as a blow to the back of the neck. Make no mistake about it; the resulting trauma is the same.

Tension and Stress

A similar reaction can result from living or working in an environment where the atmosphere is heavy with threats, insecurity, invalidation and tension. This type of mental suppression is interpreted as a threat to survival and the same restriction of circulation occurs.

We all know families and work places where there are an inordinate number of people who are sick or injured. It seems somebody is always getting hurt and sickness runs ramped. Examine the area and you'll locate someone who is creating an atmosphere of tension, invalidation and mistrust. They suppress people either overtly or covertly. The negative influence on those around this person is far reaching and devastating. Long term exposure to this person can leave you sick or crazy and can even kill you. Not only are those affected physically by virtue of the resulting constricted circulation, they are also demoralized mentally and spiritually.

The best way to deal with a person who is suppressive is by handling them so you are no longer affected by them. If all attempts to handle them fail, then you better just get away from them. Totally disconnect from them. This may seem drastic, but it's better than being sick all the time or living a life of insecurity and mistrust. Both physical injury and mental stress, of this kind, can produce inhibited circulation resulting in a myriad of illnesses, aches, pains and injury.

Long Lasting Effects of Injury

We all know someone who has had an operation of one kind or another and even though the operation was successful that person still complains of pain in that area. Or perhaps, the x-football player who injured his knee in high school, twenty years later he's hobbling around on an arthritic knee. Perhaps you know a person who was involved in an auto accident and has never completely recovered from it and is now on pain medication because the pain just won't stop. These types and many more, lasting effects of injuries account for probably 70 % of chronic aches and pains. When circulation is restricted, even a little, the tissues in that area suffer from a lack of oxygen, nutrients and other vital elements. Over time these deficiencies cause the muscles to build up lactic acid resulting in a knotting or tightening of the muscle. The muscles hurt and they never feel relaxed. The tendons and ligament and other soft tissue lose their flexibility and it hurts to move them. Chronic and continuous pain is the result.

Injuries and Arthritis

Calcium builds up on bones in areas where there is inhibited circulation. The accumulation of calcium causes a distortion of the bone structure especially around joint regions. This is one type of arthritis. Bulging knuckles, bent fingers and restricted movement are examples of arthritis.

Let's follow this along from the time of an injury. Let's say a twenty year old boy has an automobile accident and injures his knee. Even though the injury was attended to properly with the correct medical attention we find this person a year later with pains and stiffness in his knee. We find him five years later favoring that knee and now he has difficulty walking. Ten years pass and we find this fellow with arthritis in his knee and he has a great deal of difficulty bending it and he may now walk with a limp.

What's happening here? After his injury the blood vessels compressed and then they never returned to their normal size. So over time there was incomplete circulation to the knee and eventually calcium accumulated on the knee which resulted in arthritis.

What would have happened if proper attention was given to improving circulation during the healing process? If this fellow had applied a little eucalyptus liniment to his knee daily, the blood vessels would have been encouraged to function properly and he would have made a complete recovery without a long term residual incapacitating condition. I've seen this work numerous times and I'm always struck with the same conclusion that applying a little Eucalyptus liniment to the injured area should be a vital and necessary component of the healing process.

Headaches and Migraines

There are a number of other painful conditions that can result from lack of full circulation. The person who has a high pressure job suffers from headaches or even debilitating migraines. Under pressure the blood vessels in the neck and shoulder area can compress, restricting some blood flow to the surrounding muscle structure. Some of these muscles are connected to the vertebras in the neck. When these muscles tighten they can pull the vertebra down on the nerves. This shoots pain through out the head and can cause a migraine headache. The excruciating pain of a migraine headache often causes some degree of unconsciousness and thus creates a residual situation that perpetuates the condition. This same mechanism applies to what is known as tension headache. Tension and stress can cause the familiar compression of blood vessels around the neck and shoulders. Now less circulation is moving to the muscles around the head. The head muscles tighten and we now have a tension headache.

Again, eucalyptus liniment can be effective to relieve this condition. Massaging in a little eucalyptus to the back of the neck and shoulder area helps to keep circulation functioning normally. Personally, I apply a little eucalyptus liniment daily. I find by using it on my neck and shoulders, I simply don't get headaches.

Sore Feet

I've spoken with numerous people who complain about sore feet. Our feet really take a beating. I remember reading about some scientist who calculated the amount of stress the feet absorb each day. He actually calculated the amount of weight and the foot pounds of pressure encountered daily by the feet and then multiplied it out to encompass an entire lifetime. The pounds of pressure were astronomical. It's no wonder there are so many ointments, preparations, pads and potions for sore feet. Our entire body weight is continually carried on this structure, step after step for our lifetime. Feet have a big job to do. No wonder they get tired and sore.

For the most part, women complain about sore feet more often then men. It's obvious why. Those expensive and beautiful shoes that make women look so feminine are forcing their feet to operate in a fashion for which they were not intended. Those high heels that push the entire body weight to the forward part of the foot, cramming the toes, cutting off circulation and causing structural distortions must be worth the pain. Long hours on your feet in that condition can cause serious trauma. Although we can't change the fashion of the day, we can do something to help minimize the damage and the resulting pain. Massage a little eucalyptus liniment on the feet. This simple action helps to keep the blood vessels active, even in the face of constant abuse. Apply the liniment daily. Many people apply it in the morning and also at night after a hard day. The results are astonish-ing. Be good to your feet. They have a big job to do.

The Simple Truth

The simple truth of it is, when the circulation system is functioning properly sufficient nutrients, oxygen and vital elements are distributed through out the body, continually restoring it. Used and damaged cells are flushed out and the body functions optimally. When the residual effects of injuries restrict the full action of the circulation system the body sends us a signal that there is something wrong. That signal is pain. You want to do something about it before you get the pain signal. Eucalyptus can help.

The benefit of applying a little eucalyptus liniment daily are far reaching and astonishing. A simple routine of application only takes a few minutes a day and addresses a variety of common afflictions. The rewards are bountiful and neglect can be catastrophic. If more people would use this gift from nature regularly the dependency on pain medication, anti-depressants and other medications would drop dramatically. I'm looking forward to that day.

Testimonial

Suffered from severe back pain

I had severe back pain for many months. I had trouble walking and hurt all the time. I could never get comfortable whether I was lying down, sitting or standing up. I had seen four doctors, had an M.R.I., Bone Scan and many X-Rays and was prescribed pain killers and muscle relaxers. The drugs only worked to ease the pain for a few hours but left me with an upset stomach.

I saw your eucalyptus liniment at a mall and it attracted my attention because the sign said, "All Natural Pain Relief". I was willing to try anything at that point. I bought a bottle and rubbed the oil on my back and for the first time in a long while my back felt better. I continued to use it once or twice a day and the pain and the stiffness became less and less. I've been using the oil for about two years now. I put a little on my back each morning and I can walk, stand and lie down with little to no pain. At my age, 75 years old, that's a miracle. I no longer take those pain killers or muscle relaxers.

I have introduced your wonderful eucalyptus liniment to about twenty of my relatives. They all love it. Thank you for so much. It feels good to be able to enjoy life again.

Ben P.
Wilmington, Delaware

Testimonial

Sore Feet

I am a waitress and on my feet at least eight to ten hours a day. I would get home from work, take my shoes off and couldn't walk for at least an hour. Every day, it was the same thing. The pain was getting worse and I didn't know how much longer I could continue being a waitress.

I saw your display for E\eucalyptus oil at a mall. The sign said it's good for sore feet and that got my attention. The man put some on my feet and told me to take a walk and see if I notice a difference. My feet felt better right away. I use it everyday and my feet haven't felt this good in years.

Sincerely,
Judy Y.
Miami, Fla.

Testimonial

Neck pain from whip lash

I wanted you to know that since I started using your eucalyptus liniment my debilitating migraine headaches are gone. Thank you so much.

Let me back up a little. About five years ago I was involved in an auto accident. I was hit from behind and I suffered a whip lash. I've been taking medication to ease the pain in my neck and shoulders, but the pain never seemed to go away for long. The side effects of the drugs were bothering my stomach and I wanted to stop taking them. I had gone to physical therapy and they did all they could do but the pain persisted. I started getting severe migraine headaches that would leave me wiped out for an entire day or two.

I started doing some research about natural ways to reduce pain and I came across your eucalyptus liniment on the internet. I ordered a bottle about three months ago and started using it as soon as it arrived. What a relief.

I massaged it on my neck and shoulders daily and the pain was gone in days. The big surprise is my terrible migraines have not returned. I would get them once or twice a week and now in three months I have not had a single episode.

All Naturally Yours,
Susan Y.
Spokane, Washington

Testimonial

No more sore legs

A friend gave me a bottle of your eucalyptus liniment for my 60th birthday. He told me to massage it into my legs before walking my daily three mile exercise routine because it would help with circulation and my legs wouldn't get tired and stiff.

I started to use it about a month ago and I want to commend you for producing a great product. My legs do not get sore from the walk as they did in the past. I find I can complete the three mile walk with little to no strain and my legs do not throb as they did in the past.

Thanks for the help.

Pete D.
Hockessin, Delaware

Testimonial

Migraine headaches

I have suffered with migraine headaches for years. The pain would be so severe at times; all I could do was to hide in a dark room. The pain was so bad; it would cause me to throw up.

I suffered with this condition for years. I saw several doctors and was prescribed pain medication, muscle relaxers and even anti-depressants. Although these medications did help the pain somewhat, I didn't like the way they made me feel. When I was on the medication I felt like a zombie. When I didn't take them, the migraines were too much to bear. I was stuck be-tween a rock and a hard spot.

My sister was visiting me from California last summer. We were getting ready to go out to eat when I felt a migraine coming on. This was a special occasion and I didn't want to disappoint my guests by not going, so I started to take the medication. My sister said wait a minute...try this. She had a bottle of your eucalyptus oil with her and told me to give this a try. She applied some to the back of my neck and had me breath in the vapors. I felt a sudden relaxation come over me and the pain that was in the back of my head disappeared. It was amazing. We went out to diner and I felt fine all night.

The next day I ordered a bottle and this has been a best thing I could have done for myself. I use it everyday and my migraines have not returned. This has changed my life. I want you to know how pleased I am with your product. It has given my life back to me. Thank you, Thank you, Thank you!

Sincerely,

Mary S.

Media, Pa

Testimonial

On his way to a pro career

I am pursuing a career in professional basketball. My trainer suggested I use your eucalyptus liniment because of tight ligaments and tendons in one of my knees as a result of an injury I suffered a few years ago.

I was very concerned about my right knee being able to hold up under the pressure of training because this could affect my ability to play at a professional level. I applied the liniment to the knee for the first time about a month ago and felt an improvement in flexibility almost immediately. I continue to use it every time I work out and the tightness and sensitivity is gone.

This injury could have ended my dream of playing professional basketball. The dream is still alive. Thank you. When I make it to the pros, I'll send you a couple of tickets to a game.

Sincerely,
Clive O.
New York, New York

Testimonial

Arthritis in hands

I started using your eucalyptus liniment for arthritis in my hands. From the first application I could feel the difference. I have more flexibility in my fingers and the pain is greatly reduced and at times there is no pain at all. I had been taking pain pills and have stopped using them all together since I started with this oil.

I have given samples of the oil to friends of mine and they have had similar results. Many of them have ordered it from you now. This has made my life much better. Thank you.

Ralph W.
Claymont, Delaware

Chapter Five

Nature's Magical Mixture

The effectiveness of eucalyptus oil is enhanced when combined in the correct proportion with other essential oils. I've experimented with a number of mixtures and have found the following combination produces a synergistic and remarkable liniment that consistently gets the best results. The quality of the ingredients is essential to insure the liniment possesses sufficient penetrating properties. This liniment penetrates all seven layers of skin so maximum benefit can be achieved. The ingredients are as follows:

Australian Oil of Eucalyptus: There are over 600 varieties of eucalyptus. The Tasmanian Blue Gum Eucalyptus is considered the best for healing. This oil must be doubly distilled so that it contains at least 88% cineole. The grade of eucalyptus used in this liniment is crucial. A less potent grade does not have the penetrating properties. Lower grades don't have the capability to affect nerves around the blood vessels. Lower grade eucalyptus is considered cosmetic and can be found in a variety of products such as cough drops and vapor rubs. Only the most esteem Tasmanian Blue Gum Eucalyptus can be used in this liniment.

Grape Seed Oil: This is one of nature's best antioxidants. Antioxidants are important protectors of health because they neutralize the damaging effects of "free radicals". Grape seed oil has a deep penetrating property and is a natural anti-inflammatory, which assists in relieving inflammation and pain. Grape seed oil helps to carry the eucalyptus oil deep into the skin.

Aloe Vera: The Medicine Plant. The Aloe Vera plant produces at least 6 natural antiseptic agents. These antiseptics are effective against bacteria, fungus, as well as, viruses. Aloe Vera is included in this liniment because of it's effectiveness in combining with the anti-bacterial, anti-viral and anti-fungal properties of eucalyptus. Aloe Vera is also an effective pain reliever for burns and particularly sunburns.

Jojoba Oil: This oil blends well with eucalyptus oil and contains components which assist in the rejuvenation of scarred, wrinkled and otherwise damaged skin. Jojoba oil restores elasticity to dry, wrinkled skin and reduces lines and cracks. This oil is included in this liniment because it helps in the healing and mending process of the skin and restores smoothness.

Vitamin E: Just a trace of vitamin E is added to the liniment for its antioxidant effects and its unique ability to repair damaged tissue caused by harmful UV radiation.

Chapter Six

Use for Specific Ailments

Eucalyptus liniment is a light oil and comes bottled with a fine mist sprayer. Use one to seven sprays per application. If the condition is chronic or acute, apply the oil as instructed at least twice a day for the first four to five days and then at least once a day after that.

It's a Natural Vasodilator

It opens compressed blood vessels and allows more blood to flow, bringing fresh oxygen and nutrients to the cells and removes cell waste.

As circulation improves pain and inflammation will reduce.

Arthritis, Rheumatism, Fibromyalgia, Back Aches, Muscle Aches

Apply a few sprays to the area, then massage for one minute. In severe cases, after applying the liniment, use a warm compress or herb pack for ten minutes.

Sore Feet, Sprained Ankles and Knees, Tendonitis, Gout and Spurs

Rub the area all over with the liniment, then massage for about one minute. In severe cases, after massage, wrap area in warm cloth for a few minutes. You can put a little liniment in warm water and soak your feet for ten minutes. After soaking apply more liniment.

Improves Breathing and Relaxes Muscle Tension

It opens congested nasal passages and restores breathing quickly and relaxes tight muscles.

Sinus Problems, Headaches, Hay Fever, Colds, Head Congestion, Allergies and Migraines

Apply the liniment to the back of the neck and massage for 30 seconds. Apply a small amount to the temples and massage for a few seconds. Spray the liniment on a tissue, cotton ball or the palms of your hands and hold close to your nose and breath in the vapors through the nose, exhale through your mouth for sixty seconds. Then reverse the process for another sixty seconds. (The vapors may make your eyes water and cause you to cough. This is normal and is temporary.)

Asthma, Chest Congestion, Bronchitis, Laryngitis and Emphysema

Spray the liniment on a tissue, cotton ball or the palms of the hands and breathe in the vapors through the mouth, exhaling through the nose for thirty seconds. For children six years and under, inhale only once or twice.

Use in Vaporizer

Add a few drops to your vaporizer. This will make breathing easier almost immediately and will often stop coughing.

Works as an Antiseptic

It will clean the wound, stop infection and promote healing.

Cuts, Sores, Abrasions

Apply directly to affected area. If bandaged apply directly over the bandage. Saturate the bandage with the oil. It will promote healing.

Cold Sores and Skin Irritations

Apply liniment directly to affected area several times. In most cases it will stop the cold sore before it erupts through the skin.

Rashes, Insect Bites, Psoriasis, Eczema, Poison Ivy

Apply directly to the area. Repeat as necessary.

Burns and Sunburn

Immediately apply liniment to the burn and keep moist. In many cases will prevent blistering and minimizes scarring.

Acts to Naturally Soothe

Use in a Sauna

Sprinkle Eucalyptus Liniment in water and allow it to vaporize in the sauna. It's invigorating and head clearing.

Take a Eucalyptus Bath Put a capful of Eucalyptus liniment into the bath water and enjoy a soothing experience that will leave you relaxed and feeling great. You'll sleep better and have more energy.

Health for Life

Improving general circulation with the use of Eucalyptus Liniment has remarkable benefits. This simple routine performed regularly, will encourage better circulation and enhance the body's innate ability to heal and regenerate. This health maintenance routine can be done about three times a week to improve energy level, sleep more restfully and increase flexibility. Take about fifteen minutes three to four times a week and treat yourself to nature's gift of health.

All Natural Health Maintenance Routine

- ❑ Apply Eucalyptus Liniment to both feet and gently massage for about a minute on each foot. Be sure to rub the bottom of the feet and between the toes.

- ❑ Apply Eucalyptus Liniment to the neck and shoulder area and lightly massage for about a minute. If you suffer from frequent headaches, also apply a little oil to the temples and forehead. Gently massage temples for several seconds.

❑ Spray Eucalyptus Liniment on you palms and cup them over your nose. Inhale deeply through your nose and exhale out of your mouth. Do this sequence about three times then move your hands away and take three or four deep breaths through your mouth and exhale through your nose.

❑ End by massaging the liniment into your palms for a minute or so. This is very relaxing and completes the routine.

❑ A warm herbal pack placed around the neck for a few moments at the end of this routine adds to this wonderful serenity moment.

Chapter Seven

Questions and Answers

What are the ingredients of the Eucalyptus Liniment?

The Eucalyptus Liniment contains a special grade of eucalyptus oil derived from the Tasmanian Blue Gum Eucalyptus tree. This is considered the most esteem in healing because of its high concentration of cineole (the active ingredient in eucalyptus). A double distillation process insures the cineole content is at least 88%. This is combined with Grape Seed Oil, Aloe Vera, Jojoba Oil and a trace of Vitamin E.

How does it work?

This unique combination of oils can be used in a variety of ways. It is applied topically for anything from skin irritation to aches and pains caused by Arthritis. The anti viral and anti bacterial properties of the eucalyptus create a synergistic effect when blended with the other natural essential oils. When applied to the skin it is absorbed through all seven layers of skin causing the blood vessels to dilate (open, relax). When this occurs more blood can flow through the vessels bringing more oxygen and nutrients to the surrounding muscles, tissues, tendons and ligaments. This improved circulation will decrease discomfort and pain. I have found it starts to work for most people in about five minutes and will last from 5 hours to 18 hours. For people who have experienced chronic pain, I suggest they apply it twice a day for the first 4 to 5 days and then use it about once a day after that. Continued use will add circulation to the area with more and better blood flow, the body's natural ability to heal itself is enhanced.

Is it Safe?

Yes, on rare occasions certain individuals may be allergic to one of these ingredients. If this is the case, they should discontinue use. Some people I have spoken to tell me they are allergic to the eucalyptus plant but have no problem with the eucalyptus oil. This is understandable because some people have a reaction to the eucalyptus pollen, which is prolific in the plant. The pollen comes from the plant leaves. The leaves and the pollen are filtered and eliminated in the distillation process so the oil is completely free of it. This is why those who have sensitivity to the eucalyptus plant have no problem with the oil.

How can this liniment oil be effective for so many ailments?

This combination of oils addresses a variety of common issues. Viruses and bacteria play a broad role in a myriad of outer epidermal ailments. The natural antiviral and antibacterial properties focus on the root causes and therefore can be effective in their treatment.

The well documented effectiveness of Eucalyptus Oil on breathing and respiratory difficulties is beyond question. This natural oil targets the cause of these ailments and does not just attend to the symptoms.

Finally, the unique ability of this oil to act as a natural vasodilator addresses the heart of the issue when it comes to soft tissue pain and discomfort.

This combination of oils is not a panacea for every ailment and is certainly not cure all. It does help the systems of the body do what their designed to do. Therefore, the body is free to function the way it was designed and when that takes place all manner of good things can happen.

How can this one oil be effective for a variety of ailments?

Many ailments have one thing in common. They are all a result, to a greater or lesser degree, of one or more circulation problems. This oil helps to improve circulation. Additionally this strength of Eucalyptus is a natural anti-fungal, anti-viral, anti-bacterial as well as an anti-inflammatory. When you combine this strength of Eucalyptus with the other essential oils the result is a liniment that can be effective to improve health and enhance the body's natural ability to heal.

Why is circulation so important? : The circulation system carries the life-blood of the body. It has two major functions. The first is to carry oxygen, nutrition and other elements to all parts of the body. The second function is to take away waste material to be filtered and then to circulate again. As long as that system is working optimally, the body will remain generally healthy. When there is a constriction in circulation, due to injury, stress or other reasons, the full function of the circulation system is impeded and chronic ailments can occur.

How can Oil of Eucalyptus liniment help with circulation problems? : The unique properties of this type of Eucalyptus Oil caused the nerves around the blood vessels to relax; as a result, this helps the blood vessels return to there normal, unconstricted size.

With this comes better and healthier circulation and contributes to better health.

How often should I use it? : If you have an existing ailment like sinusitis, tight muscles, back pain or pain from arthritis etc. apply the oil twice a day for four to five days. After that apply once a day, or as needed.

During the cold and flu season, apply a little Eucalyptus liniment to the palms of your hands and hold your hands close to your nose and inhale. In through the nose and out through your mouth. Do this for three or four cycles at least once a day. The anti-viral and anti-bacterial properties of Eucalyptus help to proof you up against cold and flu viruses and bacteria.

Put a little Eucalyptus liniment in a bath about once a week and just soak for about twenty minutes. This is a great way to chill out. The Eucalyptus helps to relax blood vessels and the fragrance is soothing. This is a marvelous way to unwind after a hard week at work. Take the bath before you go to bed and you will enjoy a wonderful night's sleep. Its soothing action is also great for the skin.

What are other uses for the oil? : There are numerous uses. The wonderful fragrance and relaxing benefits of this unique blend lend itself to a variety of ways to enhance your personal health and well being. Listed here are just a few.

❑ **Foot massage:** We are tough on our feet, especially if we stand a lot. The muscles and blood vessels compress from the weight of our body and this can impede the normal flow of blood to muscles, tendons and ligaments. This causes feet to be tired sore and stiff. Apply Eucalyptus liniment each day to your feet and gently massage. They will feel more alive, flexible and you'll enjoy the benefits of "happy Feet". This subject is cover more thoroughly in a preceding chapter.

❑ **Massage Oil:** This is a wonderful added benefit to a relaxing massage. The fragrance will help you relax and the soothing properties of the Eucalyptus liniment will enhance circulation, adding to the overall enjoyable experience. Many massage therapists already use Eucalyptus liniment. Some people I know take a bottle with them when they get a massage and ask the therapist to use it rather than their normal massage oil.

- ❑ **Use with your shampoo:** Just one spray of Eucalyptus liniment in your hand with your shampoo and massage your scalp. It will stimulate circulation and leave your hair refreshed and feeling great.

- ❑ **In a Hot Tub:** Add a capful to the hot tub. The circulating water will massage you while the Eucalyptus Oil gently enhances this serenity moment.

- ❑ **Training and exercise:** Before working out, apply Eucalyptus liniment to the legs, back and arms. Because of improved circulation the muscles don't fatigue as fast and the recovery time is shorter.

Can Children use it? : Yes, although a very small amount is needed. We recommend not using the oil on infants because they may rub it in their eyes and mouth. You can spray a little into a vaporizer for children who are congested or have colds.

How long will the benefits of the Eucalyptus liniment last from one use? : Usually, five hours to eighteen hours. Due to the natural origin, the liniment can be applied regularly to reduce or eliminate the painful condition. This is not like a pain pill that simply hides the pain. The Eucalyptus liniment works to improve the condition that is causing the pain. It's all natural and it works by encouraging the circulation system to do what it was designed to do. To address a chronic or acute condition, the liniment can be applied at least twice a day for the first four to five days and then once a day or as needed after that.

Does the oil create heat? : No, there is nothing in the liniment that creates heat. Some people do feel some heat after they apply it. This is from their increased circulation in the area and indicates circulation was lacking in that area.

How is Eucalyptus liniment different than other topical ointments and preparations? : Most topical preparations cause a chemical reaction on the skin that produces heat. The heat has some limited benefit. However, it is very temporary and does not dilate the blood vessels to result in an overall improvement. Some people use "pain pills" which simply lowers one's awareness of the pain and have dangerous side effects. These pain pills also lower one's awareness of life without having any beneficial effect on the cause of the pain. Eucalyptus liniment improves circulation so the body's natural healing properties are enhanced. It's all natural, safe and continued use results in an improvement in the condition naturally.

After I apply the liniment, how long will the fragrance last?:

The fragrance will last about 20 minutes. So you can apply it after your shower in the morning and the fragrance will be gone before you arrive at work.

Conclusion

The intention of this book has been to enlighten the reader in the use of Eucalyptus oil. Considered by many to be the most versatile essential oil. It's applications have had a worldwide tradition of health and healing and it's benefits are now being rediscovered by modern science.

As demonstrated by many of the testimonials in this book, the benefits of eucalyptus are so remarkable that pharmacutical companies have tried to duplicate this natural compound to create a patent medication. These artificially created compounds of Eucalyptus like medication approximate the chemical composition of Eucalyptus but fail because nature is more subtle and chemicals always create a negative side effect. This attempt to duplicate Eucalyptus serves to point out the value natural Eucalyptus holds in the eyes of those who want to copy it. Natural Eucalyptus is available to everyone. A patented Eucalyptus like compound is just a substitute for the real thing.

Many of the applications mentioned in this book are hundreds of years old. They are as effective now as they were in the past. The fact that accounts of Eucalyptus use date back hundreds and hundreds of years and is now a subject of modern research further verifies it's universal appeal and effectiveness.

This book was created for educational purposes and the information is for your use. At the end of each chapter you have read testimonials from people who have used Eucalyptus liniment for their benefit. These accounts represent a relative handful of examples of what thousands of people have experienced. I personally have introduced Eucalyptus to over ten thousand individuals. It would not be difficult to fill an entire book with such accounts. The result people report covers a wide range of improvement groups. While no medical claims are made, or are ever made, about the use of Eucalyptus, I have selected testimonials which provide a broad view of persons who have benefited from its use.

This book is an offering for those who are willing to look beyond the traditional techniques to explore an even more traditional approach to health and healing. The information contained here can be used to supplement existing actions in the pursuit of optimum health and well being.

Glossary

Aborigines: The first or earliest known inhabitants of a region, natives.

Anticatarrhal: Reducing inflammation of mucous membrane in the nose and nasal passages.

Astringent: Tending to shrink mucous membrane. Checking discharge.

Aureus: Related to the ear or sense of hearing.

Catheter: Purgative, purging.

Candida: A genus of fungi, resembles yeast, occurs especially in the mouth, vagina and intestinal tract.

Decongestant: An agent that relieves congestion.

Dust Mites: Any of a large number of arachnids that live as parasites on animals, plants or dust.

Essential Oils: The droplets of oil derived from plants when compressed or distilled.

Expectorant: An agent that promotes the discharge or expulsion of mucus from the respiratory tract.

Haemophilus: A genus of bacteria associated with human respiratory infections, conjunctivitis and meningitis.

Liniment: A liquid or semi fluid preparation that is applied to the skin.

Methicillin: A semi synthetic penicillin.

Microbes: Microorganism, Germ.

Parthenogenesis: Reproduction by the development of an unfertilized seed or spore.

Pathogen: A specific causative agent of disease. Such as bacteria or virus.

Pneumonae: A disease related to the lungs.

Pyogenes: Fever producing substance.

Rhino Viruses: Any of a group of viruses that are associated with upper respiratory tract disorders.

Sinusitis: Inflammation of the sinus.

Streptococcus: A genus of parasitic bacteria.

Sudorfic: Causing or inducing sweat.

Vasodilation: Widening of the blood vessels.

Note to Reader

The contents of this book are for educational and historical purposes. Nothing listed in this book should be considered as medical advice. You should consult your health care professional for individual guidance for specific health problems. Persons with serious medical conditions should always seek professional care.

About the Author

Jack Malloy lives with his wife of 30years in Hockessin, Delaware. He has been an active naturalist for over 40 years. Their two daughters have followed in his footsteps by pursuing careers in the fields of natural health and spiritual empowerment.

Jack was the director of a very successful drug rehabilitation program where he witnessed, first hand, the devastating and demoralizing effects of both pharmaceutical and street drugs. It was at that time that he dedicated himself to the pursuit of natural solutions. He found these natural solutions, not only enhanced the body's ability to heal itself but also strengthened the individual in all areas including body, mind and spirit. This ongoing search led him in the direction of ancient remedies and much of his research is imparted in the publication for you.

Feel free to contact the author at: 302-239-2489

CPSIA information can be obtained at www.ICGtesting.com
Printed in the USA
BVOW010119120113

310302BV00002B/58/A